Family Farming Safety
Keeping Kids Safe on the Farm

Country Life Books

By Darla Noble

Mendon Cottage Books

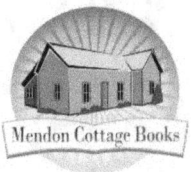

JD-Biz Publishing

Download Free Books!
http://MendonCottageBooks.com

All Rights Reserved.

No part of this publication may be reproduced in any form or by any means, including scanning, photocopying, or otherwise without prior written permission from JD-Biz Corp Copyright © 2015.

All Images owned by Darla Noble or Licensed by Fotolia and 123RF.

This book is dedicated to Danny Wilkinson, a great friend, who was killed on his family's farm in Bentley, Alberta Canada at age 15.

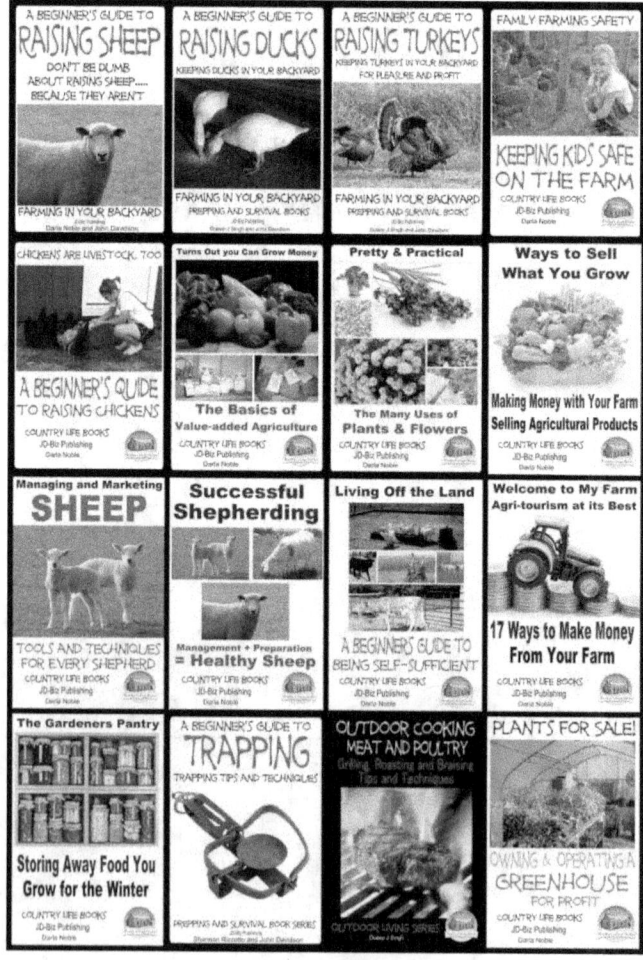

Download Free Books!
http://MendonCottageBooks.com

Table of Contents

Introduction

According to OSHA, over 300 children die each year from injuries sustained on a farm, with the overwhelming majority of these accidents being children who live on these farms (http://ehs.okstate.edu/training/oshafarm.htm) . Additionally, statistics from a number of sources all find that the number of injuries to children who live/work on family farms is over 20,000 per year.

It would be inaccurate to say that every single one of these deaths could have been prevented if better safety practices would have been in place, although, it *is* completely accurate to say that more than half of the children that die as a result of farm accidents are avoidable.

Likewise, accidents can happen even when stringent safety measures are in place, but a significant number of them could be eliminated with a few more lessons and rules in farm safety.

This book is meant to serve as both a reminder and as an educational resource for farm families with children and grandchildren as well as families whose children visit and/or work on a farm.

NOTE: Accidents happen—both non-serious and tragic accidents no one can see coming and those that are completely unavoidable despite our best efforts. This book is not meant as a guarantee against life, it is not intended to serve as legal counsel, and is not meant to serve as an endorsement for any product brand.

Chapter 1: Why is Farm Safety for Kids Such an Issue

Farm safety is an issue for kids for a number of reasons; the most prevalent of them being:

1- The term family farm means exactly what it says—the entire family works the farm. From the oldest members to the youngest, everyone has a vested interest in the farm.

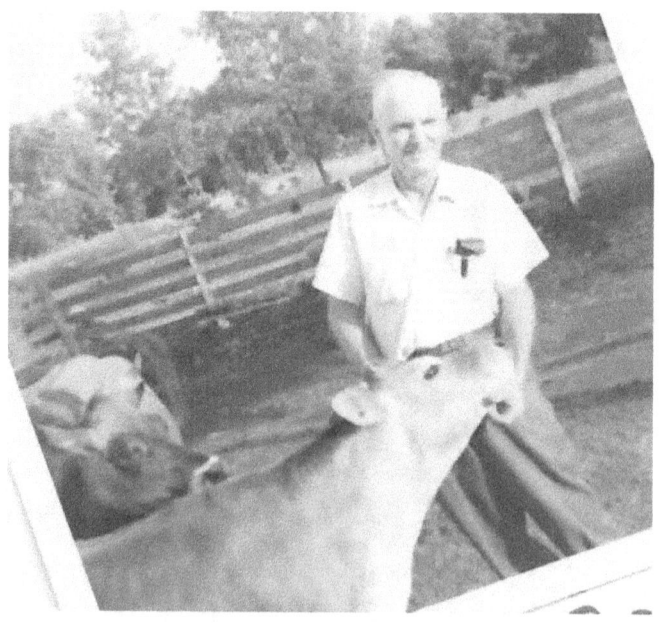

Oldest generation of a family farm

My children were the 5th generation of my family to be raised on our farm. My children sat in strollers while I milked cows by hand. They fed bottle calves, napped in playpens along the edge of a hayfield while we hauled hay, and then worked in the hay fields with us when they were old enough to do so. They helped pick garden produce and prepare it for canning, fed livestock, cleaned barn stalls and the chicken house, gathered eggs and so much more.

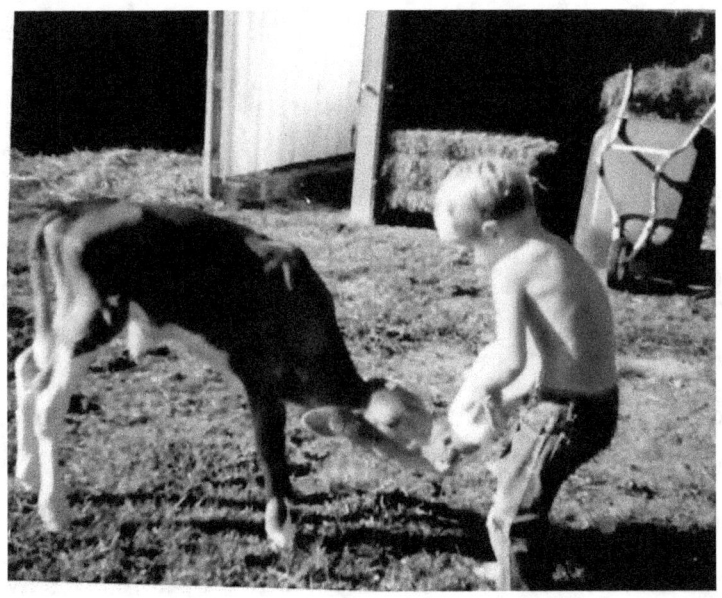

Youngest members of the family can help, too.

2- The nature of the job lends itself to greater and more safety issues. Farming is hard work that requires equipment, chemicals, livestock and other heavy materials to get the job done.

3- Kids don't understand or realize the risks and dangers involved. Even the most reliable and responsible children don't always believe they aren't invincible or indestructible. This problem is especially true when it comes to farm safety in children between the ages of 10 and 17. Children of farm families that fall within this age group are given more responsibilities than younger children. And with these added responsibilities comes greater risks due to nothing more than the rules of averages and probabilities. Case in point:

Will and Kevin were sixteen and thirteen and had grown up on their family's dairy farm. They were hard-working boys who were careful and conscientious. One cold, snowy evening, however, after milking, the boys' father sent them to feed hay to some calves while he finished up in the milk barn; something they'd done hundreds of times. William was driving the tractor and Kevin was riding beside him to get the hay when front tire of the tractor slid into a drift of snow. When it did, Kevin lost his hold; falling off directly between the front and back tires. William was unable to stop and ran over Kevin's head with the back wheel of the tractor.

This is one instance in which snow is a good thing. It cushioned Kevin and provided a padding which prevented the impact of the tire from killing him. He was airlifted to trauma center where he underwent surgery to relieve pressure on the brain and repair some damage to his eyesight.

William and Kevin didn't do anything wrong. They hadn't known the drift was there or that that tire would slip. They were, as so many other farm children are each year, a statistic of unforeseeable accidents on a farm. Thankfully, however, Kevin was extremely fortunate in the fact that forty years later he is a happy, healthy, hard-working husband, father and grandfather.

Children and farms DO go together. After all, today's farm children are the future of agriculture—which is all the more reason to do everything we can to ensure their safety today.

Chapter 2: Children and Livestock

What's a farm without livestock...unless, of course, it's a crop farm? Livestock, by their very nature, though, can be highly unpredictable. This, along with their size, weight and instincts make them a cause for many farm injuries and even a few deaths among children each year. There are several rules of safety that pertain to all forms of livestock. Let's look at these before moving on to those that are more species-specific.

Basic livestock safety rules:

*Males are easily-irritated and much more aggressive than females.

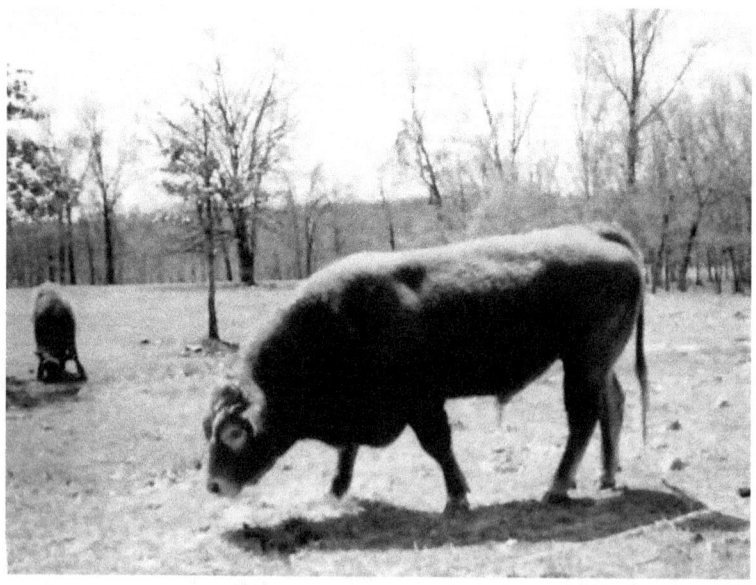

Bulls are an essential part of a herd but must be respected.

*Females with babies are instinctively protective—even to the point of aggression when they feel threatened or intruded upon.

*Livestock should always be approached from the front so they can see you coming.

*Livestock should always be approached slowly, quietly and carefully.

*When attempting to reach for or pet livestock, hold your hand out with the palm of your hand facing up and reach for the area under the chin or on the neck.

Several years ago we hosted a family reunion on our farm. Most of the people present didn't have a clue about what went on at a farm—including a cousin of mine who thought he did. He and a few others were standing in front of the pen in which our rams were housed. "Adam" was reaching his hand inside and rubbing the ram on the top of his head. The ram was butting against his hand and with each touch was growing a bit more aggressive.

This is a huge no-no. Touching a ram or bull on the head is a sign of aggression to them; one in which they will respond to aggressively. I walked over to ask him to stop, only to hear him tell the others gathered there, "See, he's really very friendly. This is just his way of saying he wants to play."

With a good amount of politeness mixed with a little bit of not-so-politeness, I quickly replied, "No, it's not. What the ram is really telling you is to back off or you'll be sorry. You should NEVER pet a ram on the head and I really need you to stop."

I then went on to explain to the others why his actions were aggressive and then showed them the proper way to pet the sheep.

*Avoid loud noises and sudden movements around livestock when trying to approach them or move them to a specific area.

*Avoid crowding an animal into a corner or tight spaces.

*Watch for signs of anger and aggression and always make sure you have a way of escape from angry livestock.

Signs of aggression to watch for when working with livestock include:

*Raised hair along the animal's back

*Snorting and/or pawing the ground

*Throwing their head

*Kicking and stomping

*Ears either laid back or pointed upward in a stiff manner

*Running/charging at you

*Bared teeth or biting

*Raised tail

*Widened eyes with whites showing

Horses

These day's horses are rarely used in the day to day operations of a farm. These day's horses are either a recreational aspect of a small farm OR they are the main or sole product of the farm. Either way, horses are a powerful animal that command our respect. For this reason, children need to be aware of the following additional safety measures when working around horses:

*Horses will kick when you stand too close to their back-end.

*Horses can and will bite.

*Horses sense fear and intimidation. Children should NEVER be left alone with a horse—even if you 'know' the horse is kid-broke.

*Horses can be impulsive and easily spooked.

When our son Zach was four, he received a small horse as a gift from a family member. The horse was gentle, easy to catch and didn't mind being ridden and handled by Zach.

One day we were outside while Zach was riding Ginger around the yard when a horsefly bit her and in an instant she was off on a dead run. She ran for quite a ways with Zach holding on for dear life and my husband running after them. Zach finally let go of his grip and rolled off of her; receiving nothing more than a bruised and scraped knee from a rock he landed on when he hit the ground.

You don't need to tell me how incredibly fortunate we were his injuries were not far worse than that.

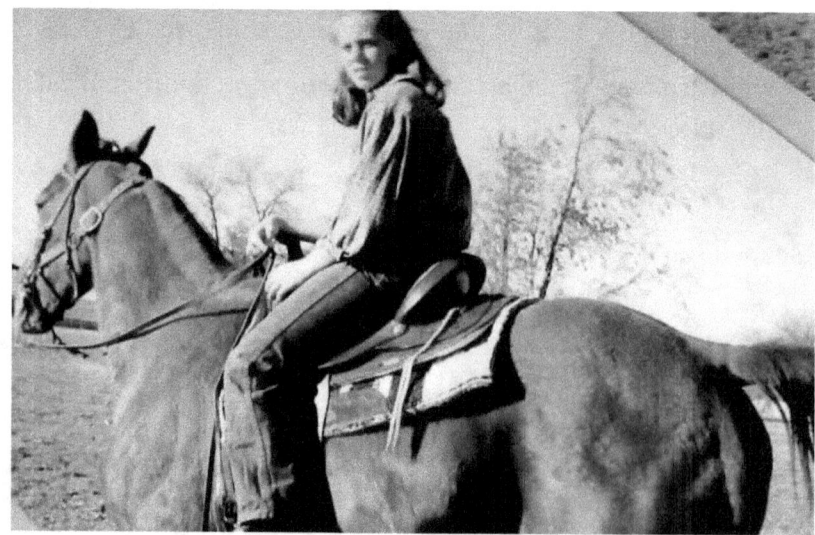

Horses can provide a great deal of pleasure to children living on a farm when treated with respect.

Chickens

Have you ever heard the term 'pecking order'? Where do you think that comes from? It comes from the fact that chickens can be sadistic little creatures that have been known to peck their fellow chickens into submission or even death in order to establish their dominance in the flock.

Nevertheless, because chickens are small, they are a great way to introduce children to farm chores and the responsibility that goes with them. Just because they are small, however, doesn't mean they aren't without their own 'set' of worries. While chickens are small in size, children need to know and adhere to the following additional safety measures when working with them:

*Never turn your back on a rooster. Getting flogged by a rooster can be very dangerous to the point of requiring stitches and leaving scars.

*Children need to know to watch for snakes and other critters that make their way into the chicken house and nesting boxes looking for eggs to eat.

*Children must be taught to wash their hands thoroughly after working with chickens, broken eggs and cleaning the chicken house to prevent salmonella and allergy and asthma problems.

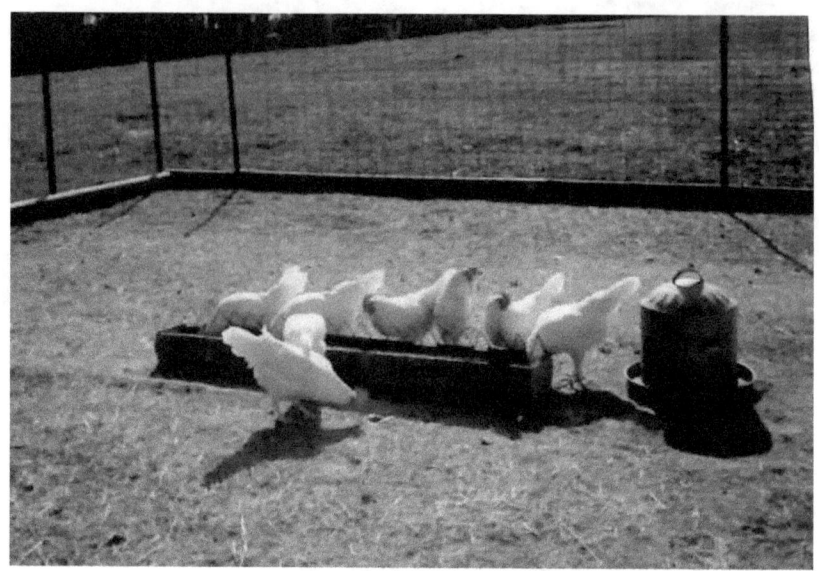

Chickens are small and a great choice

Sheep

For the most part, sheep are docile and gentle—making it easy for children to help care for and work with them…especially the lambs. They are animals, though, so like any other species of livestock, there are safety precautions which should never be ignored…especially when children are involved.

*Never turn your back on a ram. A ram's skull is extremely dense. They can easily use their heads to buckle and fold heavy gates and stock panels as if they were a piece of paper.

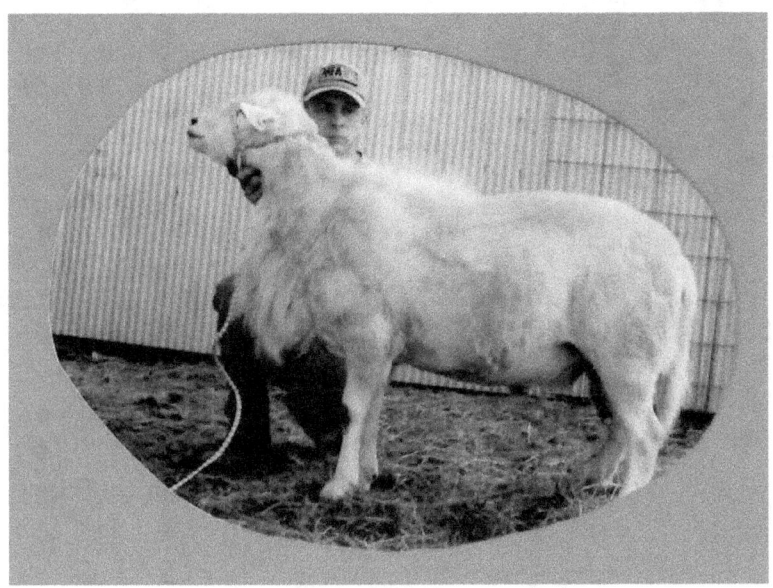

The ram, an essential part of the flock, is to be treated with respect and caution at all times.

*Never let a small child feed a flock of sheep or be in their direct path when feeding grain in a confined area. Without intentionally doing so, sheep will knock a child to the ground and run over them in order to get to their feed.

*Sheep put a great deal of trust in their shepherd. So, while you may be able to interact with a ewe and her new lambs, children who do not regularly spend time with the sheep should only be allowed to do so under your supervision.

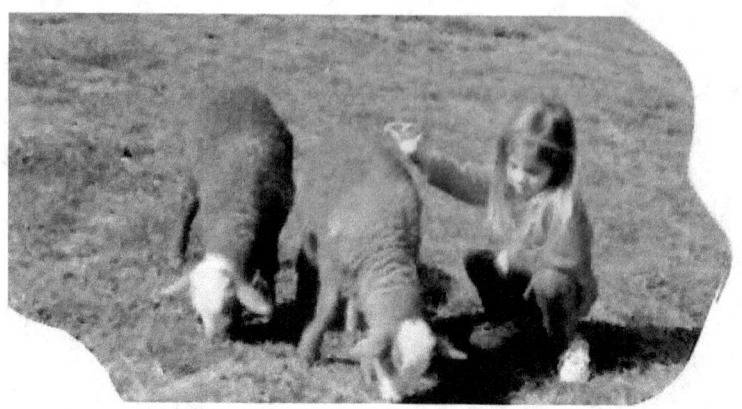

Young children who spend time with the sheep on a regular basis will be able to handle them and interact with them appropriately.

Cattle

Cattle can't help the fact that they are large, powerful animals. Parents, on the other hand, can decide whether or not to put a child at risk for being injured by the cattle on their family farm. So in addition to the basic rules of livestock safety, remember...

*Even those animals which have been worked with for showing at the fair can be unpredictable. Your children should be closely supervised when working with them.

*Do not allow children to help with loading and unloading of cattle onto a trailer. The close quarters present a huge risk for getting stepped on and/or wedged between the animal and the trailer walls.

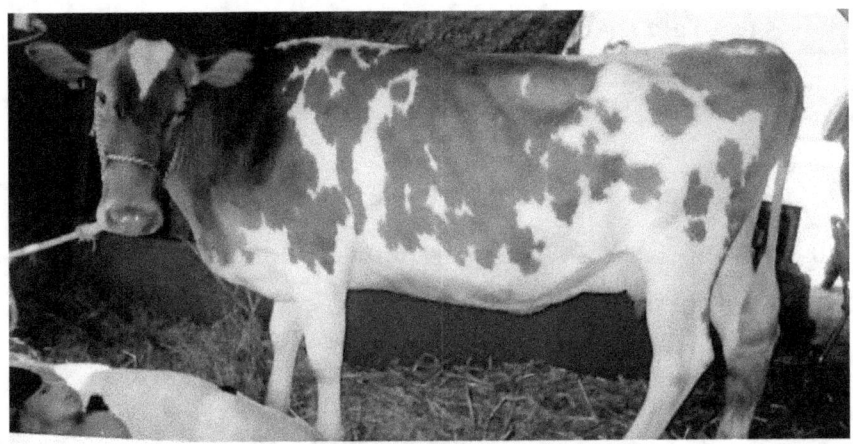

Dairy cows are generally more docile than beef cows due to the consistent daily interaction with the farmer.

*Horned cattle can and will use their horns as weapons of defense and offense. Do not allow children (even older children) to work with horned animals without close supervision.

Hogs

Hogs are usually thought to be a lazy, sloppy animal that enjoys spending its time eating and snoozing in a cool puddle of mud and muck.

Most of that is true, but when agitated, hogs can and do become aggressive and dangerous. For this reason, children should know:

*Not be in close quarters with hogs.

*A hog's teeth are sharp and strong. They can easily rip and tear through skin.

*Hogs are very protective of their babies. If a child is not normally around the hogs, they should not be allowed to interact with the babies in the presence of the sow.

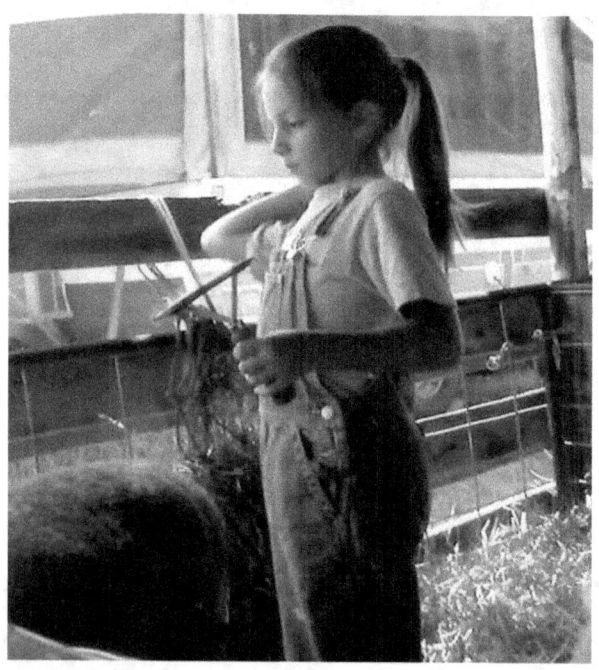

Children raised on farms gain a respect and appreciation for livestock when taught to care for them properly and safely.

Please remember this...

This book is not about taking away a child's pleasure, valuable experience, and sense of responsibility that comes in raising livestock.

It's about making these experiences as safe and productive as possible.

As a mother who raised four children on a farm, I know first-hand the value of including children in the operation of your family farm. I know that the bonds and memories made last a lifetime and will give your family something urban families will never understand or appreciate. But in order for that to happen, safety MUST be a priority.

Chapter 3: Children and Farm Machinery

Farm machinery, specifically tractors, are involved in over three-fourths of the accidents and fatalities that take place on a farm each year. ATVs are the next leading cause. In other words, we are somehow dropping the ball when it comes to kids and farm safety around farm machinery.

The keys to keeping children safe on, in and around farm machinery are really very simple. Simple, yet often ignored out of complacency and the need for extra hands to get the work done. Another common cause of farm machinery accidents among children is the lack of respect for the machine on the part of the child. NOTE: This is especially true in the instances of ATVs.

To avoid tragic and unnecessary injuries and deaths due to accidents involving farm machinery, you need to make sure the following safety rules and practices are in place:

--Machinery should be turned off when not in use

--Keys should always be kept out of the reach of children and NOT in the machine

--No child should be allowed to operate farm machinery before they have been thoroughly trained to do so and before they are old enough to have the necessary coordination to do so

--No child should be allowed to ride on a tractor or other piece of farm equipment while it is 'working' unless the child is in a seat and/or in the cab of the tractor or other piece of machinery.

--No child should be allowed to be around machinery while it is in operation. This include brush hogs, PTO shafts, balers, rakes, mowers, combines…anything that has moving parts a child can become entangled in.

The reality of the situation, though, is this…farm kids do operate farm machinery. Come hay season or harvest time, it's all hands on deck. And it's easier to have your kids drive the tractor while you feed hay off the back than the other way around.

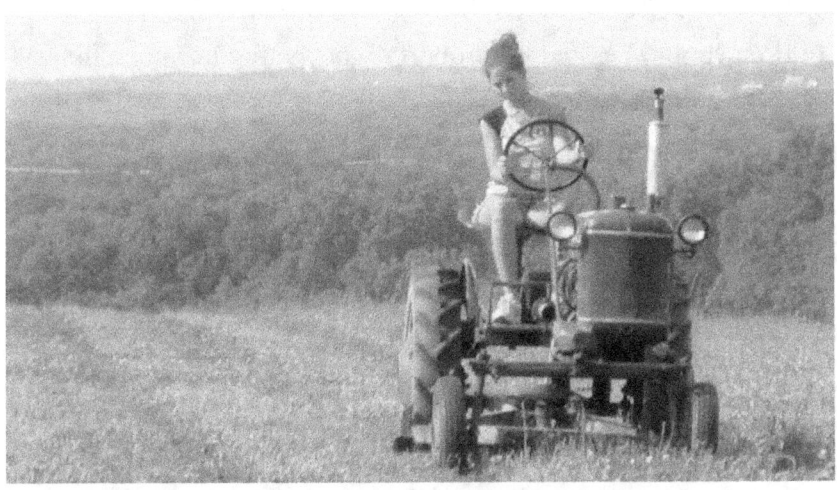

With proper teaching and supervision pre-teens and teens can safely use tractors and other farm equipment.

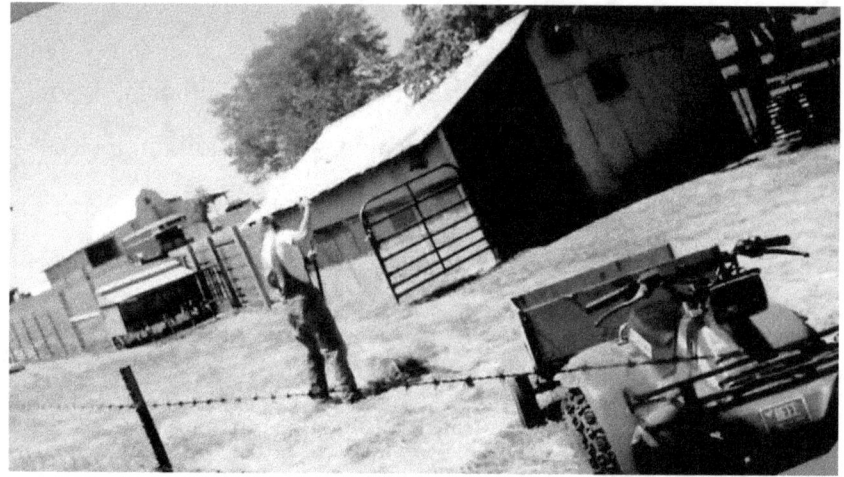

Teenagers can be trusted to operate ATVs for work and play if proper teaching and supervision has been given.

In other words, reality can be safe, too. So when your children are working with and on tractors and other pieces of farm machinery, remember these important safety tips:

--Children should be dressed properly when using farm machinery.

--Children should not be allowed to operate machinery when no one else is nearby.

--Children should not be allowed to ride or operate machinery in ravines or on embankments.

--Children should always be expected to follow the law regarding driving farm equipment on gravel roads going from field to field and should never be allowed to drive on roads and highways.

--Children should not be allowed or expected to haul trailers carrying hay or other equipment until they are old enough to be licensed drivers and trained in doing so.

Let's take a few minutes now to talk about ATVs. They are one of a farmer's best friends nowadays, as they save a lot of time and walking from one place to another. They are also valuable tools in herding livestock, hauling small loads of feed, hay and fencing and a number of other tasks. But these machines are also a great source of entertainment and fun for rural children.

Riding an ATV for fun in wide, open fields or along wooded paths is a great way to spend time with friends and family as long as it's done correctly and safely. And no, I won't leave you hanging in regards to what constitutes 'safely'. Safe ATV riding means:

You are dressed appropriately. No flip-flops, helmets are preferred or even required, safety glasses that don't cause a glare and if long pants are worn, make sure they fit tight around your ankles.

You know how to operate the machine. Riding an ATV is about a lot more than starting the engine and taking off. It's about knowing when to shift, how to balance your weight and maintaining a safe speed at all times. It's about knowing what you can and cannot ride over or ride through and about not pushing the machine beyond its limitations.

Farm tractors and other machinery are essential for operation. That's why it is equally important to make sure everyone on the farm knows and understand their purpose and their power.

Chapter 4: Children and Grains and Crops

What could possibly pose a safety risk to children when talking about grains and other crops? Actually there are quite a few risks involving these agricultural products. While injuries and deaths are not as common among farm kids in these areas, they do happen, so they are definitely worth talking about.

Hay

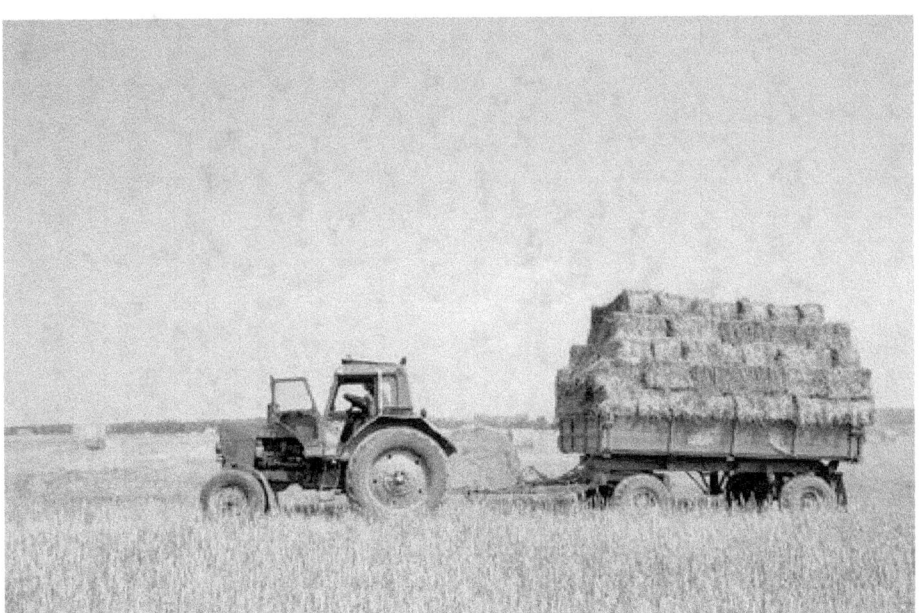

Bales of hay stacked on a trailer or in a barn always pose the risk of falling and crushing a child no matter how well they are stacked, IF a child is allowed to repeatedly climb on the hay.

Injuries can also occur when a child steps between bales of hay; causing their leg to go into the space between the rows.

Working in the hay can cause children who are asthmatic or who suffer from allergies to experience episodes of respiratory distress.

Grains

Silos and feed bins are not play places for children. Children have been severely injured and even suffocated when the grain spills or collapse on a child.

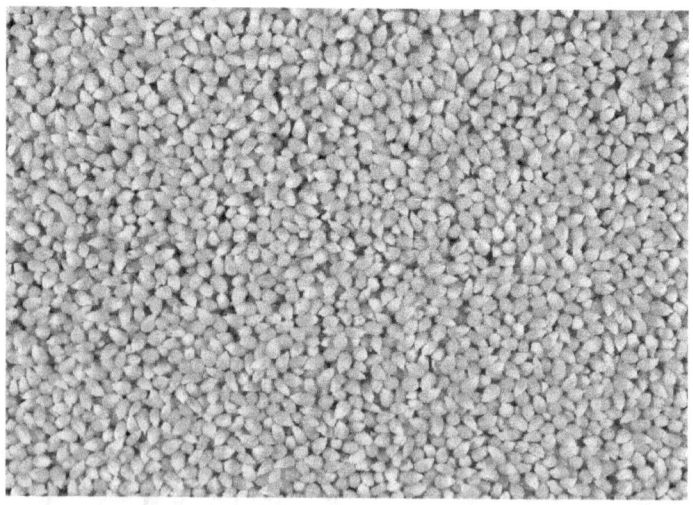

Handling bags or large buckets of feed can cause injury to a child's back or knees if they try to carry more than they are capable of handling or if they lift incorrectly.

The dust and residue from grains and other crops such as soy beans are also capable of causing respiratory distress and other allergy problems.

Chapter 5: Overlooked Farm Hazards

Livestock, machinery and crops all pose a number of hazards to children if not handled and used properly. They are not, however, the only things on the farm that can cause peril to a child on the farm.

The following is meant to serve as a reminder and a warning of the dangers 'hiding' on your farm as well as ways to prevent these things from harming your child.

Electricity

Electricity is nothing to mess around with and children should never be allowed, expected or given the opportunity to be exposed to situations in which they could receive an electric shock.

Electric lights in the barns and outbuildings should be well-grounded and should always include a shield around the bulb. Switches should be placed where there is no danger of exposure to water or risk of being disturbed or broken by animals, gates and machinery.

Electric fencing is a popular means of keeping livestock where they are supposed to be. With electric fencing, however, comes the risk of being shocked when touching the hot wires of the fence.

Receiving these little zaps of energy will do little more than cause a tingling sensation or temporary feelings of weakness when you are an adult. But a child can be burned or knocked to the ground if they touch the hot wires of the fence. Unfortunately, there is little anyone can do to prevent this from happening short of telling a child to not touch and to warn them of what will happen if they do. But we also know that the nature of a child is to do exactly what you tell them not to do in situations like this. So the best most parents can do in this case is to let them learn for themselves.

Power tools and children don't mix. Children should never be allowed to use power tools without close supervision and training on how to operate the tool safely and properly.

Parents should also keep power tools out of reach of young children and—possibly even locking them in a cabinet or tool box.

Chemicals

Farms use all sorts of chemicals depending upon the type of farm operation you have. Pesticides, herbicides, gasoline, diesel, fertilizers and livestock wormers and medications are the most common forms of chemicals a child can be exposed to. Because these substances can cause blindness, skin burns, internal burning of the lungs and other organs and possibly even death, it is imperative that you take the following safety measures in an effort to keep children safe.

*Keep all chemicals out of reach—locked away, out of sight, or on a high shelf.

*Keep a list of the chemicals you have on hand as well as treatment for external and internal exposure to the chemicals.

*Dispose of empty containers immediately upon using the chemicals. Keeping empty containers around for whatever reason is unsafe and unnecessary.

*Educate your children on the dangers of handling chemicals.

*Teach and practice proper clean-up after using chemicals. Habits such as hand-washing, cleaning up spills and wiping excess matter from the outside of the container should be done without exception.

Common hand tools

Raking out the chicken house, shoveling out barn stalls and hoeing a few weeds are usually among the first jobs a child has on the farm

Rakes, shovels, hoes and the like are all great tools to teach children how to work and are safe for children to use as long as they are coordinated enough to handle them.

Aside from teaching a child the proper usage and handling of these tools, it is important to teach a child to store these items properly. Stepping on a rake or taking a shovel to the head when you step on the handle is painful and completely unnecessary.

Chapter 6: Making Safety Fun

Cautionary. Alarming. Forewarning. Admonishment. These are the words I feel best describes the tone and message of what you've read so far.

In and of itself this isn't a bad thing—after all, farm safety for children is what this book is all about. It's just not easy to make it fun or at the very least, positive and upbeat. I hope to change that, though, with this chapter. In this chapter I want to talk about the positives of raising your children on a farm and offer information on additional resources to help you teach your children about farm safety without boring them to tears.

First of all, raising your children on the farm is one of the most valuable gifts you can give them. I say this because raising your children on the farm instills in them:

*A strong work ethic.

*The knowledge of where things come from and the work involved in making things grow.

I want to stop here and tell you a true story to illustrate just how valuable this is…

I was visiting my daughter and son in-law and granddaughter in California. We were in the commissary doing some grocery shopping when I overheard a little girl who looked to be about three, ask her mom if they could get some broccoli. The mom said yes and picked up a head of broccoli to put in their cart. As she did, the little girls asked her mom where broccoli came from. "I don't know," the mom said hatefully. It's broccoli. I guess it comes from broccoli."

I was debating on whether or not to say something to the little girl, but before I could, another lady standing nearby smiled at the little girl and said, "Broccoli is a plant, sweetie. It grows in a garden."

This just about says it all, don't you think?

*Responsibility—knowing that what they do (or don't do) matters to the rest of the family and is important to the overall operation of the farm.

*Self-worth and self-confidence that comes from accomplishing something that really matters.

*Practical skills that will prove valuable in a number of ways throughout their lifetime.

Raising your family on a farm also 'forces' you to spend time together—not just as parent/child, but as co-workers who are working toward mutual goals and successes.

Teaching your children farm safety also requires you to spend time with your child you wouldn't otherwise spend with them. This time is important but it isn't the only way to teach. There are a number of interactive resources available to help you—especially for children between the ages of three and ten. Take a look at the ones listed below and use the ones that best fit your situation.

Animal safety: http://www.farmsafetyforjustkids.org/?page_id=411

Tractor safety: http://www.farmsafetyforjustkids.org/?page_id=894

ATV safety: http://www.farmsafetyforjustkids.org/?page_id=413

Grain safety: http://www.farmsafetyforjustkids.org/?page_id=1701

Age-appropriate chores:
http://www.greeneggsandgoats.com/2014/02/farm-kids-chores.html

http://www.weedemandreap.com/age-appropriate-farm-chores/

Conclusion

Family farms are at the very core of our culture. The family farm is what made this country the outstanding nation that it is. Yes, it was the family farm—that gave the people of this country the means by which to survive. Without the grit and tenacity of farmers yesterday, today and tomorrow, we would not be able to exist.

So if you are a farm family who is raising your children to feed livestock, haul hay, hoe weeds, pick produce, gather eggs and all the other things that go with farming, be proud and thankful for the opportunity you've been given.

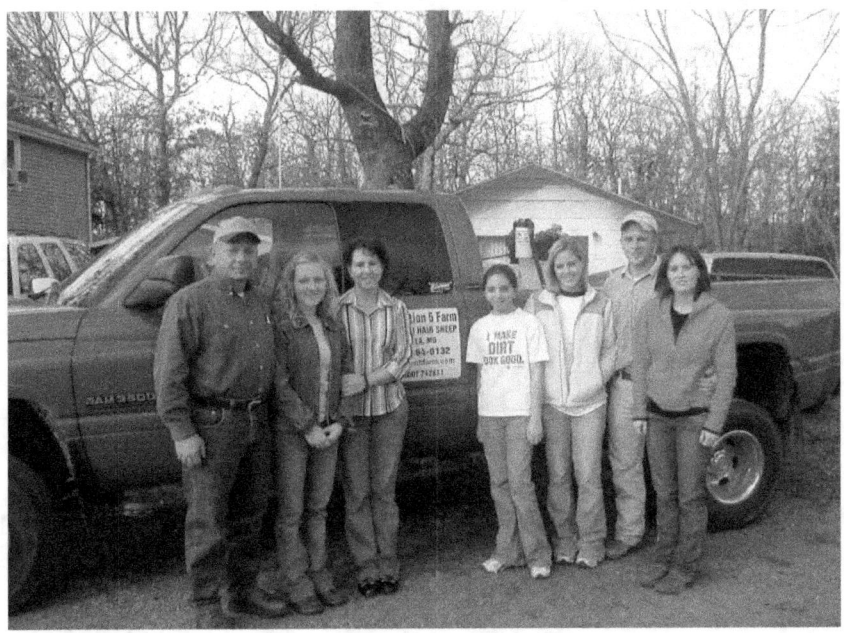

A proud farm family

Author Bio

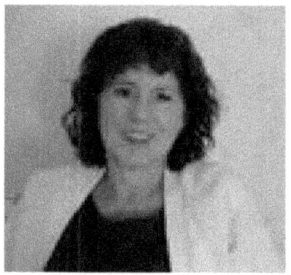

Darla Noble is a native of mid-Missouri where she lives with her Husband of thirty-three years, John. Darla's love of writing began in the fourth grade; after meeting up and coming children's author, Judy Blume, who, by the way, autographed Darla's copy of "Are you there, God...it's me, Margaret".

Darla's love for writing and family makes her work sought after in the Christian market, parenting and family resources and ghostwriting for educators and inspirational speakers.

Check out some of the other JD-Biz Publishing books

Gardening Series on Amazon

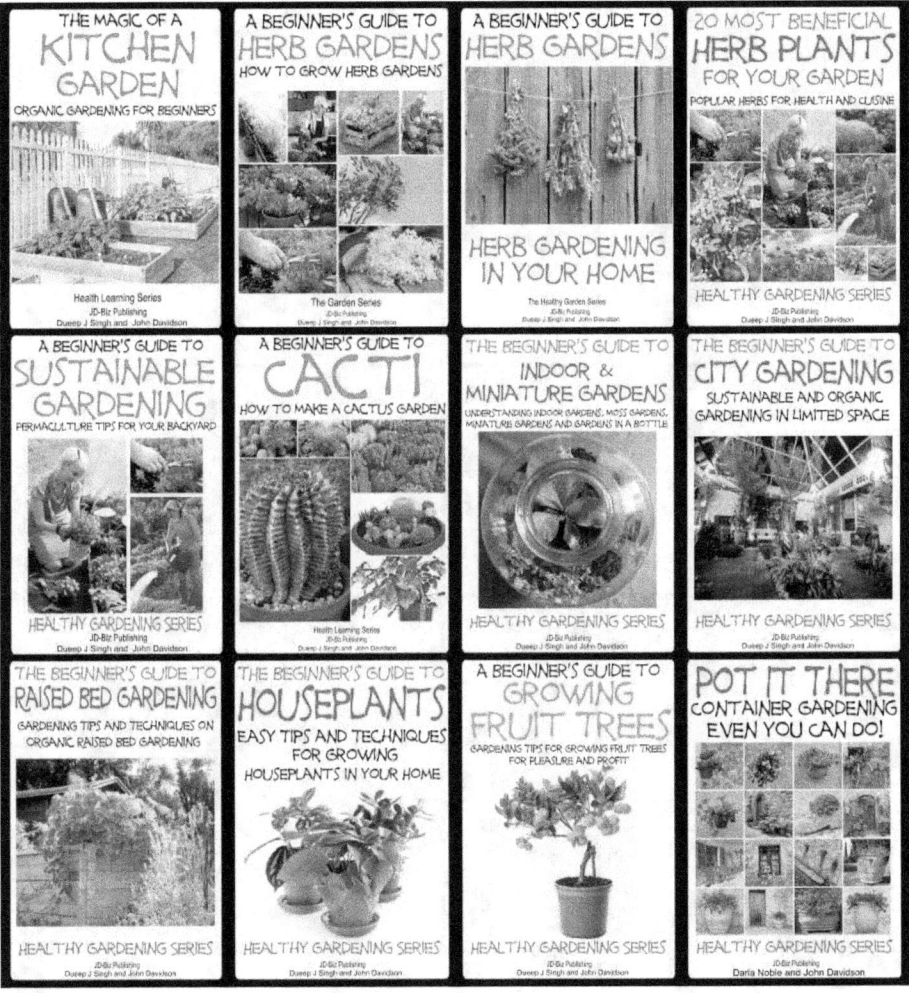

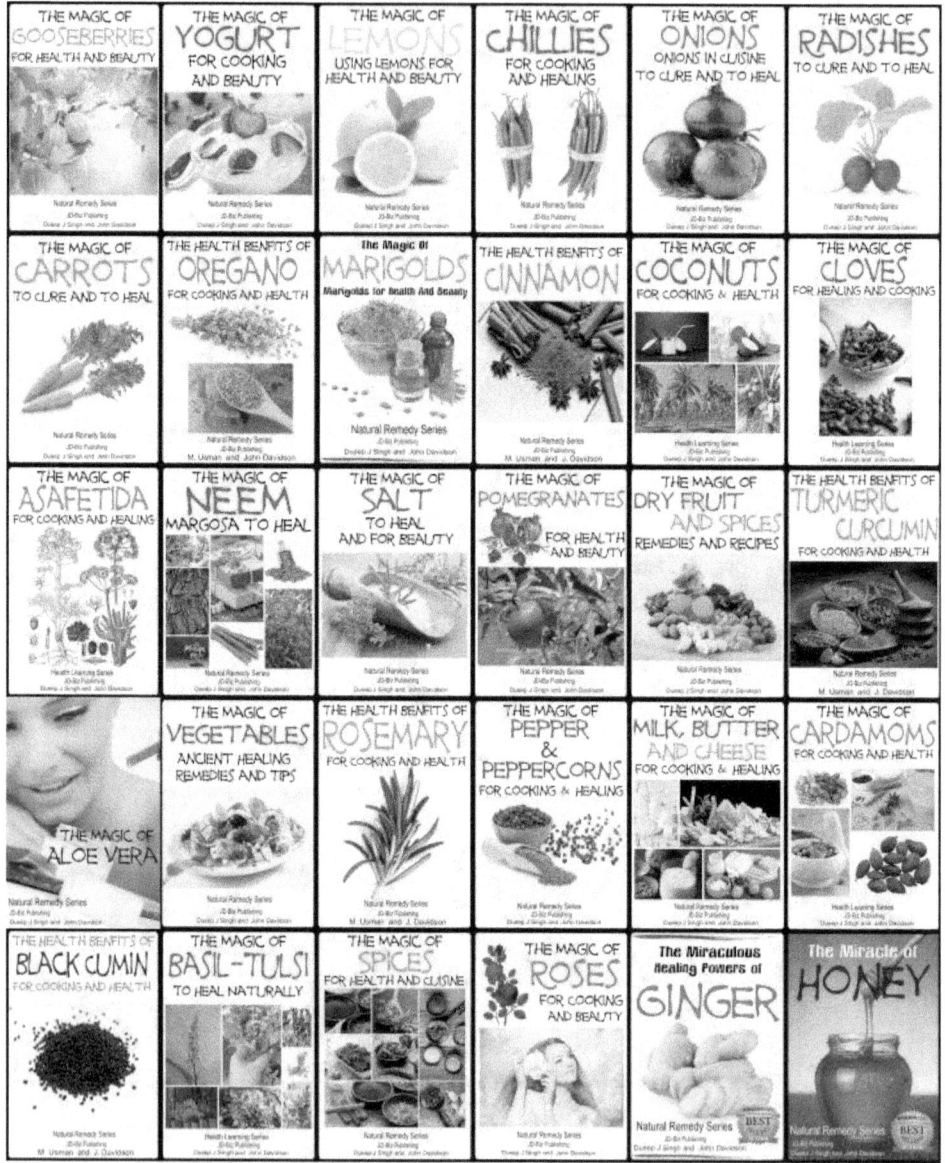

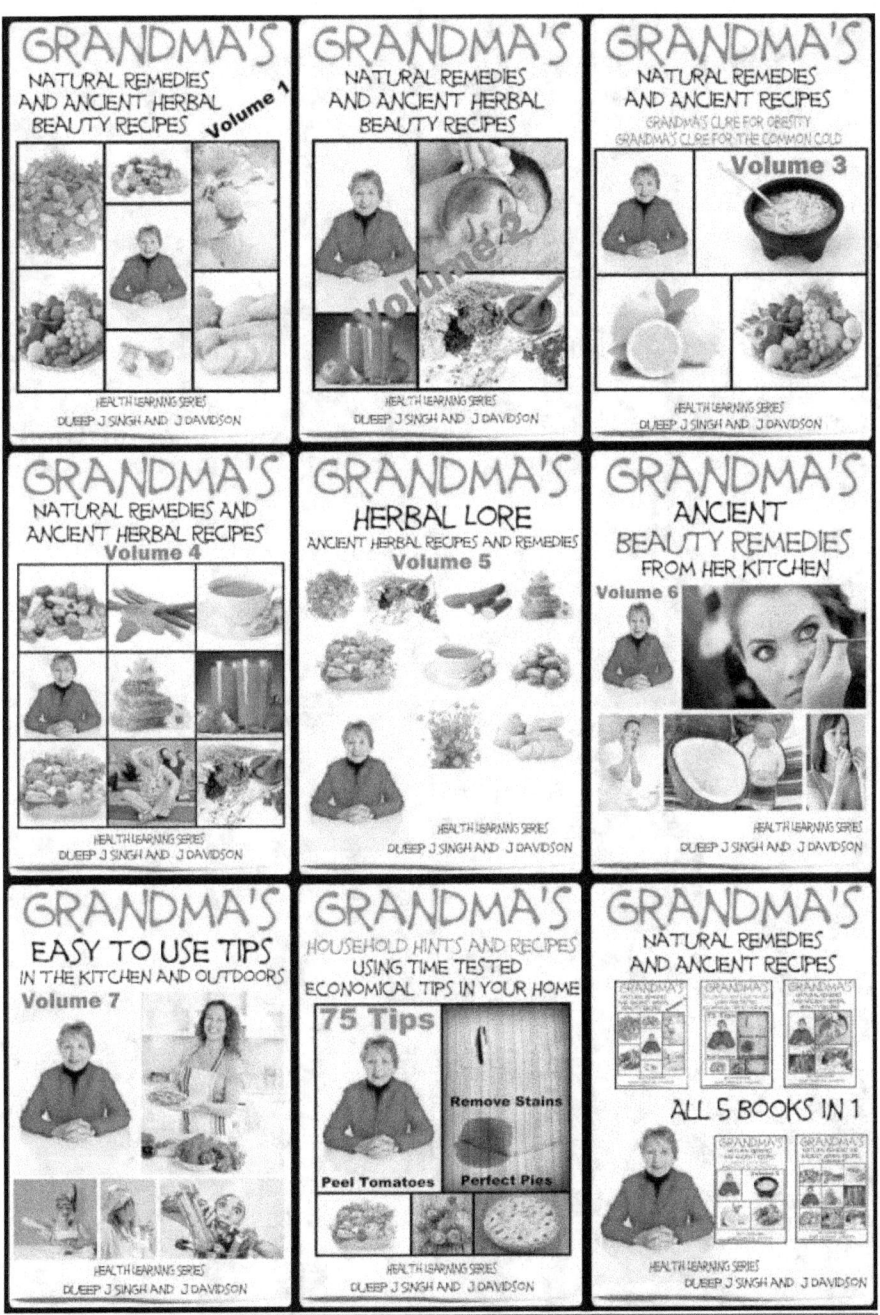

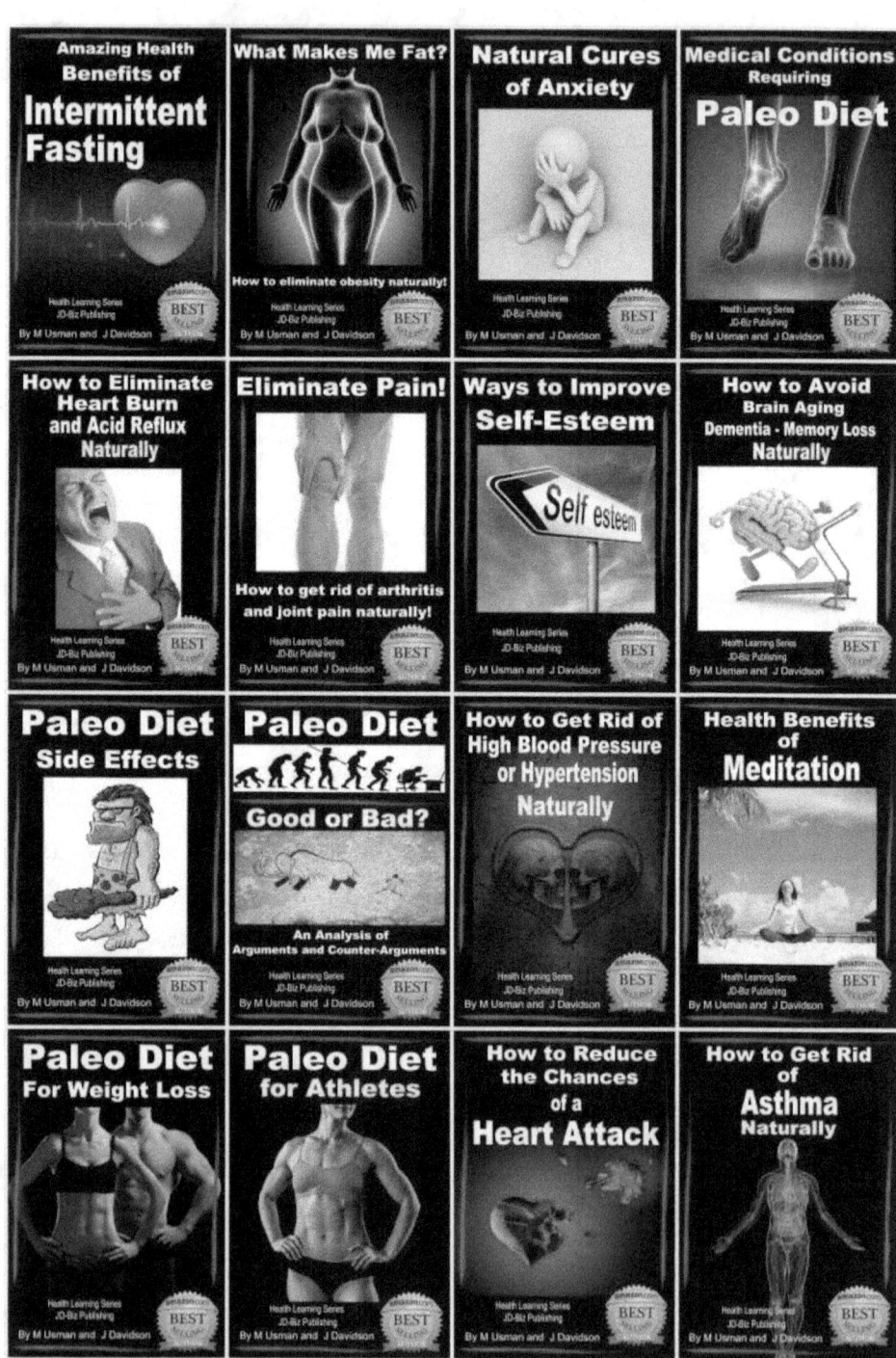

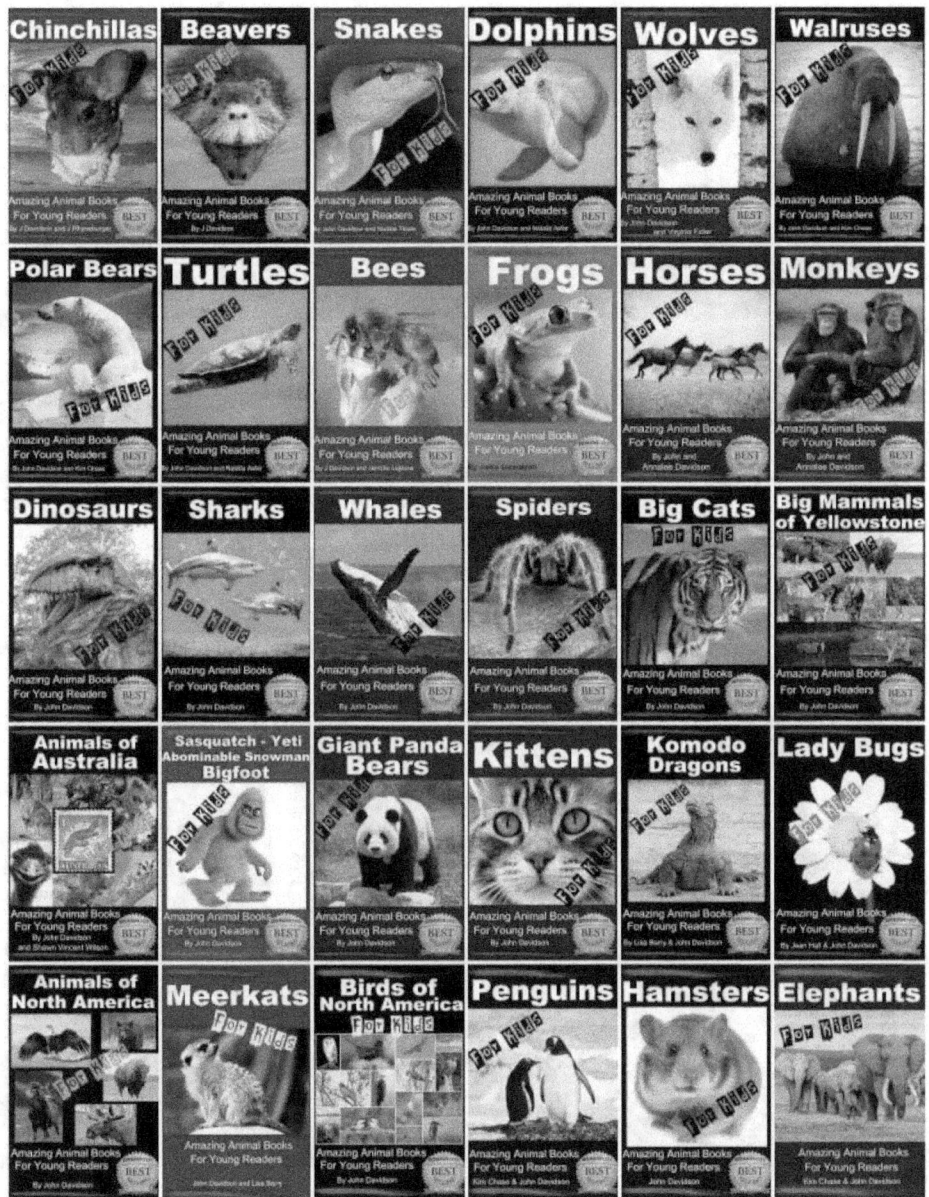

Learn To Draw Series

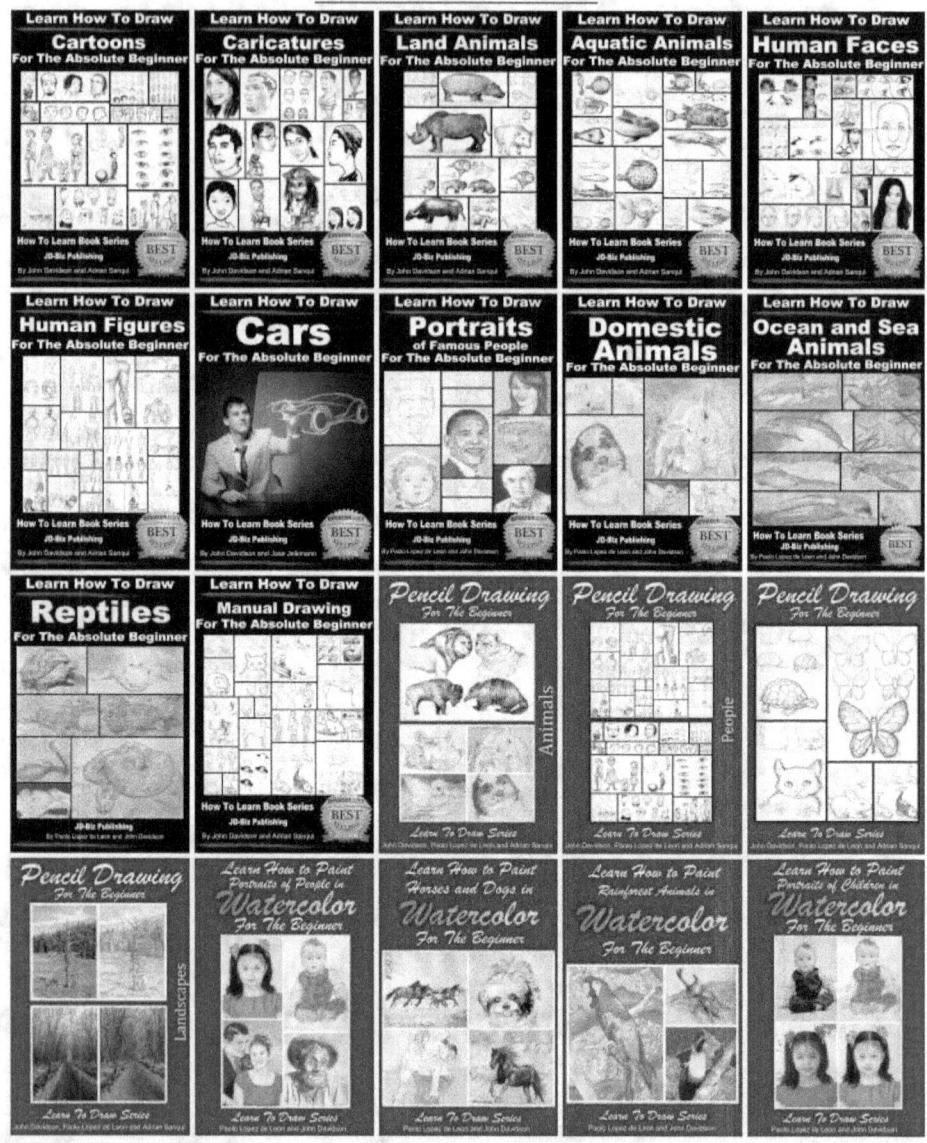

How to Build and Plan Books

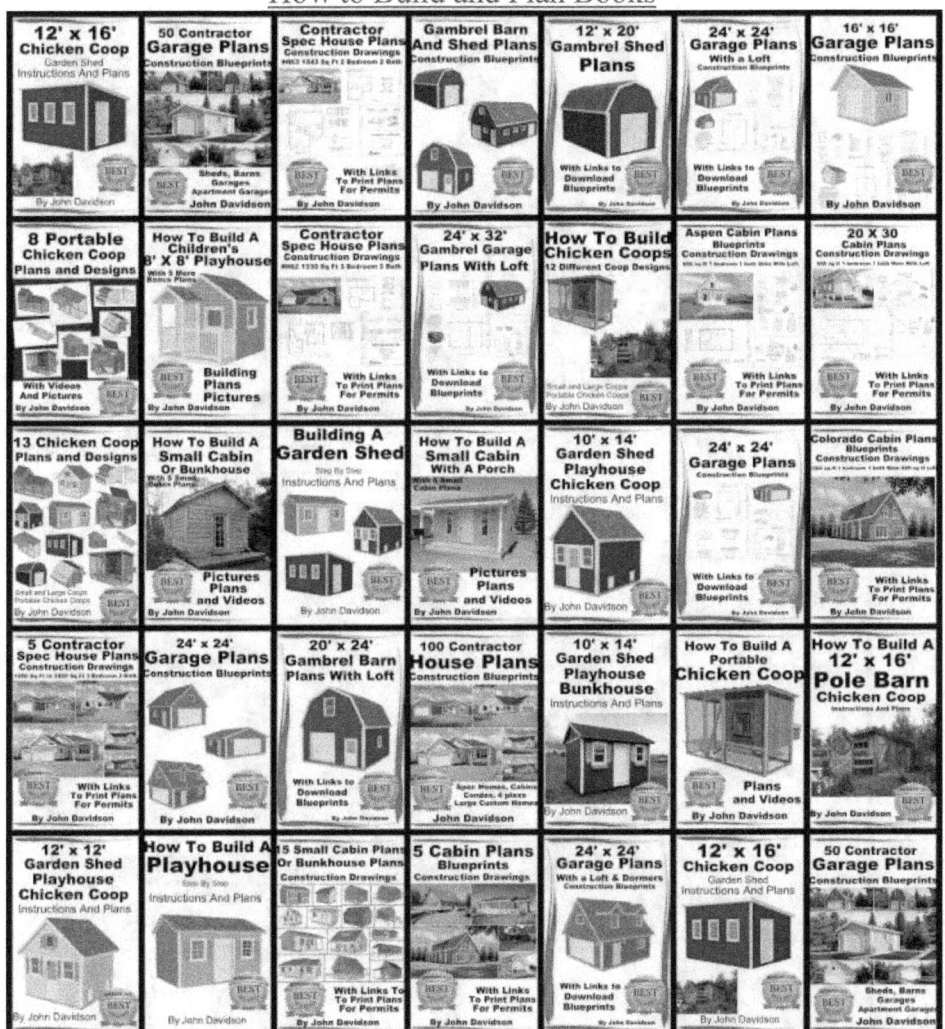

Entrepreneur Book Series

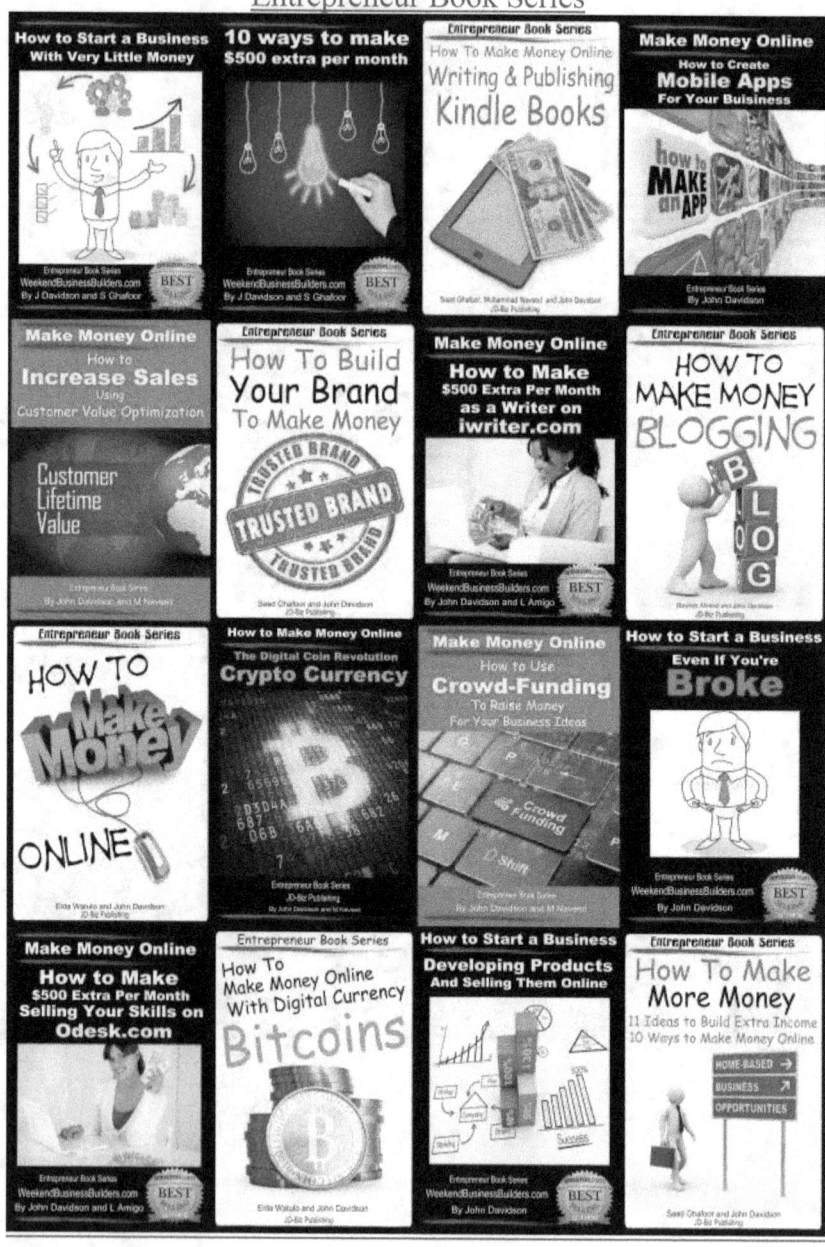

Our books are available at

1. Amazon.com

2. Barnes and Noble

3. Itunes

4. Kobo

5. Smashwords

6. Google Play Books

Download Free Books!
http://MendonCottageBooks.com

Publisher

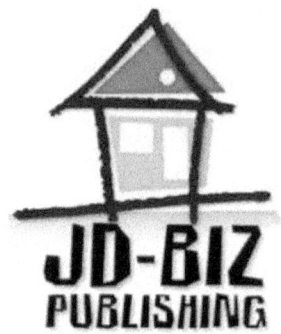

JD-Biz Corp

P O Box 374

Mendon, Utah 84325

http://www.jd-biz.com/

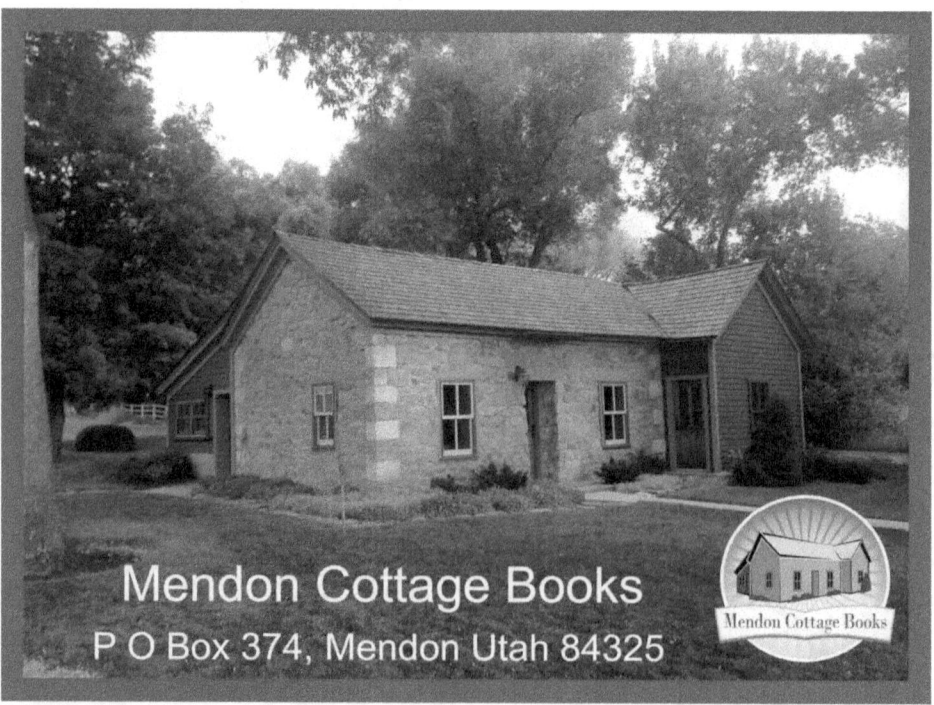

www.ingramcontent.com/pod-product-compliance
Lightning Source LLC
Chambersburg PA
CBHW071138280526
45787CB00003B/1322